PALEO SNACKS

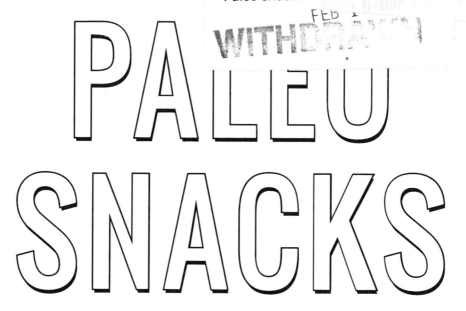

A Paleo Snack Cookbook Full of Healthy Paleo Snack Foods

|||||||||||||||||||||||||||||||||||||||||||||||||

John Chatham

CONTENTS

Chapter 3: Paleo Kids' Snacks

Chapter 4: Paleo Smoothies

Chapter 5: Paleo Sweet Snacks

Chapter 6: Low-Calorie Paleo Snacks

Section Two: The Basics of the Paleo Diet

INTRODUCTION

With its focus on whole, organic, and seasonal ingredients, the Paleo diet is not only one of the most popular diets, it's also one of the healthiest.

When it comes to Paleo meal planning, however, there is a tendency to focus entirely on entrées. But people don't live on main dishes alone. There's an entire day between breakfast and dinner and no better way to enjoy it than with healthful, delicious Paleo-friendly snacks.

With such a huge selection of tasty foods to choose from on the Paleo diet, the snacks that you can prepare are varied and satisfying. Newcomers to the Paleo diet may be surprised to learn that there are even decadently sweet treats that are perfectly in line with Paleo guidelines.

In this cookbook, you'll find something to please anyone on the Paleo diet, from sweets for the kids to meat snacks for the enthusiastic carnivore and smoothies for the hungry person on the go. There are delicious low-calorie nibbles for those trying to lose weight and snack bars to pack in school or work lunches.

During busy weekdays, it's all too easy to reach for an unhealthful snack or meal because there's no time to cook. One of the best things you can do to ensure that plenty of Paleo-friendly foods are on hand when you need them is to prepare them ahead of time. Just as spending a few hours on the weekend baking chicken breasts, roasting vegetables, or chopping a salad is time well spent, you can ensure a healthful week by preparing an array of Paleo-friendly snacks in advance.

Many of the recipes in this cookbook keep for a week or more, and many of them also freeze well. You might consider making double batches of favorite recipes so you have plenty of snacks ready to go during those especially busy weeks.

Most important, have fun trying out new recipes and Paleo-friendly versions of old favorites. The Paleo diet offers an array of delectable ingredients to choose from, so there's no reason for your diet to be boring or repetitive. With these Paleo-friendly snacks to enjoy, every day can be delicious!

Paleo Snack Recipes

PALEO SNACK BARS

No-Bake Fruit and Nut Bars

There are few snacks as beloved as chewy snack bars. These ones hit all the right notes, with a combination of nuts, coconut, honey, and dried fruit. As a bonus, you don't even have to bake to enjoy these treats! The bars keep well, so make several batches at once.

- 2 cups raw pecan halves or pieces
- 2 cups raw walnut halves or pieces
- 1/2 teaspoon sea salt
- 1/2 teaspoon cinnamon
- 1/4 teaspoon ground nutmeg
- 3 tablespoons plus 1/2 teaspoon coconut oil, melted
- 1/2 cup unsweetened shredded coconut
- 1/2 cup unsweetened dried cranberries, chopped
- 1/2 cup unsweetened dried cherries, chopped
- 1/2 cup raw honey

In a food processor or blender, grind the pecans and walnuts together until they are similar to breadcrumbs in consistency. Work in batches and be careful not to grind them too long or you will end up with pecan-walnut butter!

Pour the ground nuts into a large mixing bowl and add salt, cinnamon, and nutmeg, mixing well with your hands or a large spoon. Pour 3 tablespoons coconut oil over the mixture and blend well.

Stir in the shredded coconut, cranberries, and cherries until well mixed, then add the honey.

Line a 9 x 13–inch baking pan with aluminum foil and lightly grease the bottom and sides with 1/2 teaspoon coconut oil. Use a spoon or sturdy spatula to spread the mixture evenly into the baking pan, pressing it down firmly.

Cover with foil and let sit for 3–4 hours before cutting into bars.

Store in an airtight container for up to 1 week, or you can freeze them for up to 3 months.

Makes 1 dozen bars.

Moist and Chewy Sweet Potato Bars

Sweet potatoes are an excellent source of fiber, protein, and beta-carotene, so indulging in these bars is completely guilt-free. The bars lose a bit of their nice texture if frozen, so it's best to make just enough to last you a week.

- 2 large sweet potatoes
- 3 tablespoons hazelnut flour
- 1/4 teaspoon baking soda
- 1/4 teaspoon cream of tartar
- 1/2 teaspoon cinnamon
- 1/4 teaspoon ground nutmeg
- 1/4 teaspoon sea salt
- 1 cup unsweetened raisins
- 1/4 cup plus 1/2 teaspoon coconut oil, melted
- 1/2 cup raw honey

Preheat oven to 350 degrees F.

Poke several holes in each sweet potato with a fork and place them on a baking sheet or in a 9 x 13–inch baking pan. Bake for 45–50 minutes or until tender. Allow to cool to room temperature.

Once the potatoes have cooled, split them open and gently scoop the flesh into a large mixing bowl. Using a fork or potato masher, mash the potatoes just until there are no lumps or chunks.

In a small bowl, stir together the hazelnut flour, baking soda, and cream of tartar until well combined, then add the cinnamon, nutmeg, and salt.

Stir the dry ingredients into the mashed sweet potato, then add the raisins, 1/4 cup coconut oil, and honey.

Grease an 8 x 8–inch baking pan with 1/2 teaspoon coconut oil. Pour in the batter, smoothing it into an even layer.

Bake for 35–40 minutes or until a toothpick inserted in the center comes out clean. Allow to cool for 1 hour before cutting into bars.

Store in an airtight container in the refrigerator for up to 1 week.

Makes 1 dozen bars.

Coconut Key Lime Bars

These delicate bars will remind you of the best key lime pie, made Paleo-friendly (and extra tropical-tasting) with the use of shredded coconut and honey. They're nice and tart, and go a long way to satisfying your sweet tooth.

For the crust:
- 4 large eggs, beaten
- 1/2 cup raw honey
- 1/2 cup plus 1/2 teaspoon coconut oil, melted
- 1/4 teaspoon sea salt
- 1 cup unsweetened shredded coconut, divided

For the filling:
- 1 1/2 cups fresh key lime juice (or regular fresh lime juice)
- 9 large eggs, beaten
- 3/4 cup raw honey
- 1/4 teaspoon sea salt
- 3/4 cup coconut oil, melted

Make the crust:

Preheat oven to 350 degrees F.

In a large bowl, stir the eggs, honey, 1/2 cup coconut oil, and salt until completely combined.

In a blender or food processor, grind 1/2 cup of the shredded coconut until it resembles flour and stir it into the egg mixture. Add the remaining shredded coconut and stir until combined.

Grease the bottom and sides of a 9 x 13–inch pan with 1/2 teaspoon coconut oil, and smooth the crust mixture into the pan.

Bake for 15–17 minutes until light golden brown. Set aside to cool.

Make the filling:

Whisk together the key lime juice, eggs, honey, and salt in a large bowl until well blended.

Pour into a deep saucepan over medium heat. Whisking constantly, slowly add the coconut oil.

Continue whisking and cook until the mixture thickens enough to coat the back of a spoon. Remove from heat and pour the filling into the cooled crust. Refrigerate for 4 hours before cutting into bars.

Store in the refrigerator for up to 1 week, keeping them chilled until ready to eat. These bars don't freeze well.

Makes 1 dozen bars.

Banana Walnut Bars

Nothing is quite as comforting on a cool morning or evening as a slice of warm banana bread. This recipe brings you that familiar flavor in a dense, moist bar with a delightfully crunchy walnut topping. The secret to their deliciously moist texture is unsweetened applesauce. These freeze well, so make plenty.

- 4 large overripe bananas, mashed
- 1 cup unsweetened applesauce
- 2 eggs, beaten
- 1/2 cup plus 1 teaspoon coconut oil, melted
- 1 teaspoon pure vanilla extract
- 1 cup coconut flour
- 1 teaspoon baking soda
- 1/4 teaspoon sea salt
- 3/4 cup chopped raw walnuts

Preheat oven to 375 degrees F.

In a large mixing bowl, combine the bananas, applesauce, eggs, 1/2 cup coconut oil, and vanilla. Either in a stand mixer or with a hand mixer, beat on low speed for about 1 minute, until well blended. Add the coconut flour, baking soda, and salt, and beat for 1–2 minutes until the dry ingredients are incorporated.

Grease the bottom and sides of a 9 x 13–inch baking pan with 1 teaspoon coconut oil. Pour the batter into the prepared pan, smoothing until even, and top with the chopped walnuts.

Bake for 35–40 minutes or until a toothpick inserted in the center comes out clean. Cool to room temperature before cutting into bars.

Store wrapped in plastic wrap in the refrigerator for up to 1 week. To freeze, wrap in plastic wrap and then aluminum foil. The bars will keep in the freezer for up to 3 months.

Makes 1 dozen bars.

Banana-Cocoa Swirl Bars

For chocolate lovers, getting a cocoa fix can be a bit of a challenge on the Paleo diet. These bars give you a satisfying dose of chocolate flavor without straying from the diet and without being too sweet. They're also very pretty, so bring them out for company or take them along to a potluck.

- 6 medium, overripe bananas, mashed
- 2 large eggs, beaten
- 1 tablespoon plus 1 teaspoon coconut oil, melted
- 1 teaspoon pure vanilla extract
- 1 cup coconut flour
- 1 teaspoon baking soda
- 1/2 teaspoon ground allspice
- 2 tablespoons unsweetened cocoa powder

Preheat oven to 350 degrees F.

In a large mixing bowl, combine the bananas, eggs, 1 tablespoon coconut oil, and vanilla, and stir with a spoon until smooth.

In another bowl, combine the coconut flour, baking soda, and allspice. Gradually mix the dry ingredients into the banana mixture, until just incorporated.

Pour half of the batter back into your flour bowl and add the cocoa powder, mixing well.

Grease a 9 x 13–inch pan with 1 teaspoon coconut oil. Pour half of the cocoa-banana mixture into the baking pan, smoothing to form an even layer.

Pour the plain banana mixture on top, smoothing again. Dollop the remaining cocoa-banana mixture evenly over the plain, and swirl them together with a toothpick or the tip of a knife.

Bake for 40–45 minutes or until a toothpick inserted in the center comes out clean. Allow to cool to room temperature before cutting into bars.

Store wrapped in plastic wrap in the refrigerator for up to 1 week. To freeze, wrap in plastic wrap and then aluminum foil. The bars will keep in the freezer for up to 3 months.

Makes 1 dozen bars.

Pumpkin Spice Bars

If pumpkin pie is your favorite part of Thanksgiving, or if warm, spicy pumpkin bread is your top comfort food, these bars will hit the spot. They are wonderfully dense and moist and loaded with fragrant spices, just as pumpkin treats should be. They freeze very well, so make a few batches at once and you'll be ready for the holiday season!

- 1 (28-ounce) can pumpkin puree (not pumpkin pie filling)
- 2 large eggs, beaten
- 1 tablespoon plus 1 teaspoon coconut oil, melted
- 1 teaspoon cinnamon
- 1/2 teaspoon ground ginger
- 1/2 teaspoon ground nutmeg
- 1/2 teaspoon ground allspice
- 1 cup coconut flour
- 1 teaspoon baking soda
- 1/2 cup unsweetened raisins
- 1/2 cup chopped raw walnuts

Preheat oven to 350 degrees F.

In a large bowl, combine the pumpkin puree, eggs, 1 tablespoon coconut oil, cinnamon, ginger, nutmeg, and allspice. Whisk together until well blended.

In a small bowl or measuring cup, combine the coconut flour and baking soda, then stir into the pumpkin mixture, until just blended. Stir in the raisins and walnuts.

Grease a 9 x 13–inch pan with 1 teaspoon coconut oil. Pour the batter into the pan, smoothing the top.

Bake for 45–50 minutes or until a toothpick inserted in the center comes out clean. Allow to cool to room temperature before cutting into bars.

Store wrapped in plastic wrap in the refrigerator for up to 1 week. To freeze, wrap in plastic wrap and then aluminum foil. The bars will keep in the freezer for up to 3 months.

Makes 1 dozen bars.

(2)

PALEO PROTEIN SNACKS

Spicy-Sweet Chicken on a Stick

These chicken skewers are marinated in a spicy, slightly sweet sauce that makes them impossible to resist. They're a satisfying snack anytime, but they also make a terrific appetizer for parties. To make them into a meal, remove the skewers and chop the chicken into a fresh green salad.

- 1 teaspoon coriander
- 1 teaspoon ground chili powder
- 1/2 teaspoon onion powder
- 1/2 teaspoon garlic powder
- 1/2 teaspoon sea salt
- 1/2 teaspoon freshly ground black pepper

- 4 large (about 2 pounds total) boneless, skinless chicken breasts
- 1/2 cup olive oil
- 2 tablespoons raw honey
- 12 bamboo skewers, cut in half and soaked in water 30 minutes

In a small bowl, combine the coriander, chili powder, onion powder, garlic powder, salt, and pepper until well mixed.

Rub the seasoning mixture all over both sides of the chicken breasts and place on a plate. Cover with foil or plastic wrap and allow to sit in the refrigerator for at least 1 hour.

Meanwhile, heat the olive oil and honey in a small saucepan over low heat, stirring frequently, until the honey is just melted. Set aside and allow to cool to room temperature.

Remove the chicken from the refrigerator and cut each breast lengthwise into 5–6 strips. Place the strips in a Ziploc-type plastic bag. Pour the olive oil–honey mixture into the bag, seal, and shake.

Place the chicken in the refrigerator overnight or for at least 4 hours.

Place your oven's broiler rack about 6 inches from the broiler element and turn on the broiler. Line a baking sheet with aluminum foil.

Thread each chicken strip onto a bamboo skewer by weaving it in a ribbon-like fashion, being sure to make at least 2–3 punctures with the stick.

Place the skewers onto the baking sheet and broil for 5 minutes. Turn each skewer over and broil for another 4–5 minutes or until the chicken is cooked through.

To serve, place the chicken on a platter, skewer-side out for easy grabbing, and serve warm or at room temperature.

Makes about 20 to 24 skewers.

Marinated Zucchini-Salmon Bites

Who needs crackers when these tangy zucchini slices make such a fresh and tasty foundation for smoked salmon! This is a perfect appetizer for summer barbecues and elegant dinner parties alike.

- 1 cup apple cider vinegar
- 1 teaspoon pickling spices
- 2 medium zucchini, cut into 1/2-inch slices (about 2 dozen total)
- 1 Hass avocado, mashed (about 3/4 cup)
- 2 teaspoons fresh lemon juice
- 6 ounces smoked salmon, thinly sliced
- 2 tablespoons poppy seeds

Bring the apple cider vinegar and pickling spices to a simmer in a medium saucepan over medium heat.

Remove from heat and add the zucchini slices. Allow them to soak for 20 minutes, then remove to paper towels to dry.

In a small bowl, combine the avocado and lemon juice, mixing well.

Cut the sliced salmon into about 2 dozen (2-inch) strips.

Pat the zucchini slices dry and spread each slice with avocado, top with a piece of salmon, and sprinkle with poppy seeds.

Serve the bites arranged on a platter at room temperature or chilled.

The marinated zucchini slices will keep overnight in the refrigerator, covered with plastic wrap. Assemble right before serving, so the avocado doesn't brown.

Makes about 2 dozen pieces.

Hawaiian-Style Beef Jerky

Meat jerkies are a Paleo mainstay and a delicious one at that. Jerky can be made with a wide array of flavorings, is extremely portable, and is very easy to make in either the oven or a dehydrator. This recipe has the added benefit of stretching your meat budget since it uses less-expensive cuts.

- 2 pounds grass-fed flank steak or top round steak
- 1 teaspoon sea salt
- 1/2 teaspoon freshly ground black pepper
- 1 cup unsweetened pineapple juice
- 2 teaspoons grated ginger (or jarred chopped ginger)
- 2 teaspoons chopped fresh garlic

Place the steak in the freezer for about 30 minutes to make it easier to slice.

Slice the steak across the grain into 1/2-inch-thick slices. Season with salt and pepper, then put the meat slices in a gallon-sized Ziploc-type plastic bag.

Combine the pineapple juice, ginger, and garlic, and pour into the bag. Seal and shake to coat the meat evenly.

Marinate in the refrigerator 6–8 hours or overnight, turning the bag a few times to distribute the marinade evenly.

Line a baking sheet with a double layer of paper towels. Remove the slices of meat from the bag one at a time, shaking them gently to remove excess marinade, and place them on the paper towels. (The meat slices should be in a single layer. If you run out of room, use a second baking sheet.) Cover the slices with another double layer of paper towels and press down to squeeze out excess moisture. Allow to sit for 20 minutes, then slide the paper towels (along with the meat) off the baking sheet.

Position oven racks at the center and bottom. Line the bottom rack with aluminum foil to catch drips.

Heat the oven to "warm" (about 160–165 degrees F). If using a dehydrator, set it to 135 degrees F.

Line the baking sheet(s) with aluminum foil for easier cleanup, and place wire cooling racks onto the baking sheet(s).

Arrange the meat slices in a single layer on the wire racks, spaced so that the slices do not touch each other. (This allows for proper airflow.) If using a dehydrator, simply layer the strips onto the trays without the pieces touching.

Place the baking sheet(s) on the center rack in the oven and dry for 2–3 hours or until the meat is somewhat cracked and looks a bit stringy. It should not be overly dry; this jerky is meant to be moist and chewy. Open the oven door 3–4 times during drying to allow moisture to escape. If using a dehydrator, your drying time will be 3–4 hours.

Store the jerky in a Ziploc-type plastic bag in the refrigerator for up to 2 weeks. Do not freeze.

Makes about 1 1/2 pounds.

Savory Venison Jerky

Venison can be very inexpensive if deer are hunted in your area (or if you have a hunter in the family). It's a naturally lean protein and is ideal for jerky. Drying time will vary depending on the leanness of the meat, so check the jerky frequently to prevent overdrying.

- 2 pounds venison shoulder or loin, visible fat removed
- 1 tablespoon paprika
- 1 teaspoon sea salt
- 1 teaspoon freshly ground black pepper
- 1 cup unsweetened apple juice

Place the venison in the freezer for about 30 minutes to make it easier to slice.

Slice the meat across the grain into 1/2-inch-thick slices. Season with paprika, salt, and pepper, then put the slices in a gallon-sized Ziploc-type plastic bag.

Pour the apple juice into the bag. Seal and shake to coat the meat evenly.

Marinate in the refrigerator 6–8 hours or overnight, turning the bag a few times to distribute the marinade evenly.

Line a baking sheet with a double layer of paper towels. Remove the slices of meat one at a time from the bag, shaking them gently to remove excess marinade, and place them on the paper towels. (The meat slices should be in a single layer. If you run out of room, use a second baking sheet.) Cover the slices with another double layer of paper towels and press down to squeeze out excess moisture. Allow to sit for 20 minutes, then slide the paper towels (along with the meat) off the baking sheet.

Position oven racks at the center and bottom. Line the bottom rack with aluminum foil to catch drips.

Heat the oven to "warm" (about 160–165 degrees F). If using a dehydrator, set it to 135 degrees F.

Line the baking sheet(s) with aluminum foil for easier cleanup, and place wire cooling racks onto the baking sheet(s).

Arrange the meat slices in a single layer on the wire racks, spaced so that the slices do not touch each other. (This allows for proper airflow.) If using a dehydrator, simply layer the strips onto the trays without the pieces touching.

Place the baking sheet(s) on the center rack in the oven and dry for 2–3 hours or until the meat is somewhat cracked and looks a bit stringy. It should not be overly dry; this jerky is meant to be moist and chewy. Open the oven door 3–4 times during drying to allow moisture to escape. If using a dehydrator, your drying time will be 3–4 hours.

Store the jerky in a Ziploc-type plastic bag in the refrigerator for up to 2 weeks. Do not freeze.

Makes about 1 1/2 pounds.

Chicken-Cherry Wraps with Paleo Mayo

These wraps are quite versatile, as they are equally satisfying as a snack or light lunch, and you can also use the filling as a topper for celery sticks or cucumber slices or to stuff avocado halves.

For the Paleo mayo:
- Yolk of 1 large egg, beaten
- 2 tablespoons fresh lemon juice
- 3/4 cup light olive oil
- 1/2 teaspoon sea salt

For the chicken spread:
- 3 large cooked chicken breasts, chopped (about 2 cups)
- 2 stalks celery, thinly sliced
- 1 small sweet onion, chopped
- 1/2 cup unsweetened dried cherries, roughly chopped
- 1/4 cup chopped raw pecans
- 2 tablespoons Paleo mayo
- 1/2 teaspoon sea salt
- 1/4 teaspoon freshly ground black pepper
- 6 leaves romaine lettuce

Make the Paleo mayo:

In a small saucepan, combine the egg yolk and lemon juice, and place over low heat.

Whisking constantly, cook until the mixture is just thick enough to coat the back of a spoon. Pour into a shallow dish and refrigerate for about 20 minutes to cool.

Pour the mixture into a medium-sized mixing bowl and very slowly whisk in the olive oil, about 1 tablespoon at a time. The mixture will begin to turn opaque and creamy in color. Whisk until all the oil is incorporated, then whisk in the salt.

Store in an airtight plastic container or jar in the refrigerator for up to 3 days.

Makes 1 cup.

Make the chicken spread:

In a medium mixing bowl, combine the chicken, celery, onion, cherries, and pecans, and stir well. Stir in the Paleo mayo until well blended, season with salt and pepper, and stir again.

Place about 1/4 cup of chicken spread onto the wide end of a lettuce leaf, and roll up like a burrito. Repeat with remaining lettuce leaves.

Makes 6 wraps, or cut in half for 1 dozen snack bites.

Paleo-Happy Deviled Eggs

Deviled eggs are a must-have when it comes to summer picnics and barbecues. This recipe uses homemade Paleo mayo to make it completely Paleo-friendly. It's unlikely you'll have leftovers, but if you do, chop them up for a quick egg salad lettuce wrap.

- 1 dozen hard-boiled large eggs, peeled
- 1/4 cup diced sweet onion
- 1 teaspoon mustard
- 2 tablespoons Paleo mayo (see Chicken-Cherry Wraps with Paleo Mayo)
- 1 teaspoon chopped fresh dill
- 1/2 teaspoon sea salt
- 1/4 teaspoon freshly ground black pepper
- Paprika for sprinkling

Cut each egg in half lengthwise. Remove the yolks and place them in a medium-sized mixing bowl. Set the whites aside on a platter. If any whites break or tear, chop them up and add them to the yolks.

Use a fork to mash the yolks until they are evenly crumbled.

Add the onion, mustard, Paleo mayo, dill, salt, and pepper, and stir until well blended.

Scoop about 1 tablespoon of filling into each egg-white half, and sprinkle paprika over all.

Cover and refrigerate for about 1 hour before serving.

These will keep in an airtight container in the fridge for 1 day.

Makes about 2 dozen.

Spicy Cucumber-Tuna Bites

When you need a satisfying and protein-rich snack, this spicy tuna salad atop refreshing cucumber slices fills you up without weighing you down. This recipe makes extra tuna salad, perfect for lunchtime wraps or sandwiches.

- 2 (6-ounce) cans salt-free tuna packed in water
- 1 tart apple (such as Granny Smith or Braeburn)
- 1/4 cup finely chopped sweet onion
- 1/4 cup finely chopped celery
- 4 medium cucumbers, peeled
- 1 teaspoon mild curry powder
- 1/2 teaspoon sea salt
- 1/4 teaspoon freshly ground black pepper
- 2 tablespoons Paleo mayo (see Chicken-Cherry Wraps with Paleo Mayo)

Drain the tuna very well and place it in a medium-sized mixing bowl.

Core, peel, and finely chop the apple.

Combine the tuna, apple, onion, and celery, and stir well.

Add the curry powder, salt, and pepper, and stir with a fork until well blended. Mix in the Paleo mayo. Cover and refrigerate for 1 hour to allow the flavors to develop.

Cut the ends off the cucumbers and use a fork to carve lines lengthwise through the skin. Slice the cucumbers into 1/2-inch-thick slices (about 4 dozen).

Spread each cucumber slice with about 2 teaspoons of tuna mixture. Arrange on a platter to serve.

The filling will keep in an airtight container in the fridge for up to 3 days.

Makes about 4 dozen pieces.

Broiled Sardines

Sardines are an excellent source of protein, omega-3s, and calcium, especially if eaten with the bones. But even if you love tinned sardines, they get boring pretty quickly on their own. This recipe adds fresh flavor to this inexpensive and healthful fish, and transforms it into something completely new.

- 1 1/2 teaspoons light olive oil, divided
- 4 (3.75-ounce) cans sardines packed in water
- 1/4 cup finely chopped red onion
- 1 teaspoon paprika
- 1/2 teaspoon garlic powder
- 1/2 teaspoon sea salt
- 1/4 teaspoon freshly ground black pepper
- 2 tablespoons finely chopped fresh basil

Place your oven's broiler rack about 6 inches from the broiler element and turn on the broiler.

Line a small baking pan with aluminum foil and grease with 1/2 teaspoon olive oil. Place the sardines in the pan in a single layer (their sides will be touching).

Scatter the chopped onion over all, then drizzle with 1 teaspoon olive oil.

Sprinkle the sardines with the paprika, garlic powder, salt, and pepper. Top with chopped basil.

Broil for 1–2 minutes, just until the fish turns lightly golden. Serve warm.

Makes 4 servings.

3

PALEO KIDS' SNACKS

Nutty Carob Apple Slices

Kids love making these treats almost as much as they love eating them. There's no cooking involved, so they're a great way to get little ones involved in the kitchen. Parents will appreciate the fact that they satisfy kids' cravings for a sweet snack and are good for them, too.

- 4 crisp apples, such as Gala or Fuji
- 1 tablespoon fresh lemon juice
- 1/2 cup almond butter
- 1 tablespoon carob powder
- 1 tablespoon raw honey
- 1/4 teaspoon pure vanilla extract
- 1/4 cup chopped raw walnuts

Core and slice the apples into wedges (about 6–8 slices each), leaving the peel on.

Place the apple slices in a bowl and toss with the lemon juice.

In a blender or food processor, combine the almond butter, carob powder, honey, and vanilla, and blend just until the carob and honey are well incorporated.

Drain the apple slices and pat dry with paper towels.

Spread one side of each apple slice with the almond butter mixture, then sprinkle generously with chopped walnuts. Serve immediately or chill until ready to eat.

(To use for school lunches, soak desired portion of apple slices overnight in the lemon juice and store the spread separately in an airtight container. In the morning, simply spread the almond butter mixture onto the apple slices, top with walnuts, and pack in a single layer in an airtight container.)

Makes about 16 pieces.

Frozen Coco-Nut Banana Pops

Kids love ice-cream treats, but they don't make for a healthful snack (nor are they Paleo-friendly). Satisfy your kids' ice cream cravings with these frozen banana pops coated in nut butter and toasted coconut. They're ideal for kids' parties, too.

- 4 large green-tipped bananas (just ripe)
- 8 Popsicle sticks
- 1/2 cup almond butter
- 2 tablespoons raw honey
- 1 teaspoon cocoa powder
- 1 cup unsweetened, toasted coconut flakes

Peel the bananas and cut in half crosswise. Insert a Popsicle stick through the cut end of each banana half.

In a blender or food processor, combine the almond butter, honey, and cocoa powder, and blend until smooth. Spoon the mixture out onto one end of a cutting board. Mound the toasted coconut on the other end of the cutting board.

Line a rectangular, airtight plastic container with waxed paper, and place it on the counter next to the coconut.

Roll each banana pop in the nut butter mixture to coat all sides, then roll it in the coconut. Place the pops in the plastic container, alternating ends so they don't touch.

Cover and freeze for at least 2 hours before serving. They will keep in the freezer up to 2 days.

Makes 8 servings.

Lunch Box Granola Mix

This kid-friendly granola mix does double duty as a nutritious snack to tuck into lunch boxes or as a filling breakfast, topped with almond milk. This recipe makes a lot, but it'll be gone in no time.

- 1 cup raw pecan halves
- 1 cup sliced raw almonds
- 1 cup raw pumpkin seeds
- 1/2 cup unsweetened dried cherries, roughly chopped
- 1/2 cup unsweetened dried apricots, roughly chopped
- 1 cup unsweetened golden raisins

- 2 tablespoons raw honey
- 1 teaspoon pure vanilla extract
- 2 tablespoons coconut oil, warmed
- 1/2 teaspoon sea salt
- 1/2 teaspoon cinnamon

Preheat oven to 275 degrees F.

In a large mixing bowl, combine the pecans, almonds, pumpkin seeds, cherries, apricots, and raisins.

Stir the honey and vanilla into the coconut oil until the honey melts. Add the salt and cinnamon, stir well, and pour over the granola mixture. Toss the granola thoroughly with a spoon or clean hands (hands work best).

Line a baking sheet with aluminum foil and pour the granola onto it in a thin layer.

Bake for 15–20 minutes, just until golden brown. Allow it to cool completely on the baking sheet before storing.

Store in an airtight container at room temperature for up to 2 weeks.

Makes about 5 cups.

Chicken Fingers with Paleo Ranch Dip

Kids love chicken strips and ranch dressing, but neither one is Paleo friendly in its traditional form. This quick and easy recipe is a nutritious take on the fast-food classic. Pack a larger portion in an insulated bag for a school lunch—it's sure to be a hit.

For the Paleo ranch dip:

- 1 cup unsweetened coconut milk
- 1 cup Paleo mayo (see Chicken-Cherry Wraps with Paleo Mayo)
- 1/2 teaspoon garlic powder
- 1/2 teaspoon onion powder
- 1/2 teaspoon sea salt
- 1/2 cup chopped fresh dill
- 1/4 cup chopped fresh parsley

For the chicken fingers:

- 4 small boneless, skinless chicken breasts
- 2 large eggs, beaten
- 1 tablespoon unsweetened coconut milk
- 1/2 cup coconut flour
- 1/2 teaspoon paprika
- 1/2 teaspoon sea salt
- 1/2 teaspoon garlic powder
- 1/4 cup unsweetened coconut flakes
- 3 teaspoons olive oil, divided

Make the Paleo ranch dip:

In a medium-sized mixing bowl, combine the coconut milk, Paleo mayo, garlic powder, onion powder, and salt, and mix well.

Stir in the fresh herbs, cover, and refrigerate for at least 1 hour.

Makes 2 cups.

Make the chicken fingers:

Preheat the oven to 375 degrees F.

Cut the chicken breasts lengthwise into 1-inch-thick strips, and cut longer strips in half (if needed) to make each strip about 3 inches long.

In a large bowl, beat the egg yolks and coconut milk together with a fork, then add the chicken strips, tossing to coat.

In a medium bowl, combine the coconut flour, paprika, salt, and garlic powder, and whisk until well combined. Stir in the coconut flakes.

Line a baking sheet with aluminum foil. Grease the foil with 1 teaspoon olive oil.

Remove the chicken strips from the egg mixture one at a time, tapping to remove excess egg, and dredge in the flour mixture before placing on the baking sheet.

Drizzle the remaining olive oil over all, and bake for 15–20 minutes or until juices run clear when the chicken is pierced with a fork.

Serve warm with a small dish of Paleo ranch dip alongside.

Makes 4 servings.

Grilled Fruit Kebobs

It's easy enough to get kids to eat an apple or a pear, but if you want to give them something special, this recipe is just the ticket. Oven grilling brings out the natural sweetness of the fruit and caramelizes the honey, making these kebobs extra delicious.

- 1/2 teaspoon coconut oil
- 1/2 cup fresh pineapple chunks
- 1/2 cup fresh watermelon chunks
- 1/2 cup fresh cantaloupe chunks
- 1/2 cup green seedless grapes
- 8 bamboo skewers soaked in water for 30 minutes
- 1/4 cup raw honey
- 1/2 teaspoon sea salt

Place your oven's broiler rack about 6 inches from the broiler element and turn on the broiler. Line a baking sheet with aluminum foil and grease the foil with coconut oil.

Thread the fruits onto the bamboo skewers, alternating them as you like. (Kids love to help with this part.) Lay the skewers in a single layer on the baking sheet.

Microwave the honey in a small dish for 15 seconds, then pour it over the fruit skewers. Sprinkle the sea salt over all.

Broil for 2 minutes on each side, until just golden. Allow to cool at least 10 minutes before serving, as the fruit will be very hot.

Makes 8 servings.

Oven-Fried Sweet Potato Chips

When you start feeding your kids a healthful diet, potato chips and other salty deep-fried snacks are among the hardest to give up. Luckily, these sweet potato chips have just enough salt to satisfy cravings, and oven frying in olive oil provides a healthier crunch.

- 4 large sweet potatoes, peeled and very thinly sliced (a food processor slicing attachment or mandoline works best)
- 2 tablespoons olive oil
- 1 teaspoon sea salt
- 1/2 teaspoon freshly ground black pepper

Preheat oven to 300 degrees F.

In a large mixing bowl, combine the sweet potato slices, olive oil, salt, and pepper, and toss well to coat. (Clean hands work best.)

Line two large baking sheets with aluminum foil.

Spread the chips onto the baking sheets in a single layer and bake for about 40–50 minutes or until very dry and crisp.

Allow the chips to cool to room temperature before serving.

Store the chips in an airtight container for up to 1 week.

Makes about 4 cups.

PALEO SMOOTHIES

Paleo Piña Colada

This tropical smoothie is like an island vacation in a glass. As creamy and rich as it is, it's perfect for dessert, but it's healthful enough to serve as a quick breakfast on the go. Kids especially love this smoothie, so try it on the little ones as a cooling summer snack.

- 1 cup unsweetened coconut milk
- 1 (10-ounce) can unsweetened chopped pineapple, with juice
- 1 teaspoon raw honey
- 1/2 teaspoon pure vanilla extract
- 1/2 cup unsweetened coconut flakes
- 6 ice cubes
- Pineapple chunks, for garnish

In a blender, combine the coconut milk, pineapple with juice, honey, and vanilla. Blend on high until smooth.

Add the coconut flakes and ice cubes and blend on high just until the ice is crushed and the mixture is thick and smooth.

To serve, pour into tall glasses, and garnish with pineapple chunks on toothpicks, if desired.

Makes 4 servings.

Nutty Cocoa-Banana Smoothie

This restorative shake is excellent pre- or post-workout. The almond butter lends a nice richness, and the banana provides a healthful dose of carbs and potassium. To make it extra thick, freeze the mixture for an hour or so, then blend it again until smooth before serving.

- 1 cup plain, unsweetened almond milk
- 1 large ripe banana, peeled and broken into pieces
- 4 tablespoons almond butter
- 1/2 teaspoon pure vanilla extract
- 2 teaspoons cocoa powder
- 1 teaspoon raw honey
- 6 ice cubes

In a blender, combine the almond milk, banana, almond butter, vanilla, cocoa powder, and honey. Blend on high just until the bananas and cocoa are well incorporated.

Add the ice cubes and blend on high until the ice is crushed and the mixture is smooth and thick.

To serve, pour into 2 tall glasses and drink immediately.

Makes 2 servings.

Summertime Peach Smoothie

This recipe is a great way to enjoy peaches when they're at their most abundant, nutritious, and flavorful. You can substitute frozen, unthawed peaches if the fresh fruit is not in season. This is also an excellent way to use up peaches that have become a bit overripe or bruised.

- 2 ripe peaches, peeled and sliced (about 1 1/2 cups)
- 1 cup plain, unsweetened almond milk
- 2 tablespoons unsweetened orange juice
- 1/2 teaspoon pure vanilla extract
- 6 ice cubes
- 1/4 teaspoon ground nutmeg

In a blender, combine the peaches, almond milk, orange juice, and vanilla. Blend on high until the peaches are incorporated and smooth.

Add the ice cubes and blend on high until smooth and thick.

To serve, pour into 2 tall glasses and sprinkle with nutmeg.

Makes 2 servings.

Orange Dream Smoothie

If you're a fan of the orange sherbet–vanilla ice cream combo, you'll love this smoothie. It's equally delicious as a snack or dessert, and kids are especially enthusiastic about its resemblance to the ice-cream truck classic.

- 1 cup plain, unsweetened almond milk
- 3 tablespoons unsweetened frozen orange juice concentrate
- 1 teaspoon pure vanilla extract
- 1 teaspoon raw honey
- 6 ice cubes

In a blender, combine the almond milk, orange juice concentrate, vanilla, and honey. Blend on high until smooth.

Add the ice cubes and blend on high until thick and creamy.

Pour into 2 glasses and serve immediately.

Makes 2 serving.

Cocoa-Hazelnut Smoothie

When you have the urge to reach for that jar of chocolate-hazelnut spread, which is loaded with sugar and bad fats, reach for this smoothie instead. You'll get your fix, without compromising your healthful diet. Feel free to use almond butter instead (adding 1/2 teaspoon almond extract) if you prefer almond flavor to hazelnut.

- 1 cup plain, unsweetened almond milk, divided
- 1/4 cup hazelnut butter
- 2 tablespoons plus 1/2 teaspoon cocoa powder, divided

- 2 teaspoons raw honey
- 6 ice cubes

In a small bowl or measuring cup, combine 4 tablespoons almond milk with the hazelnut butter and stir with a fork until the mixture is pourable.

In a blender, combine the remaining almond milk, the hazelnut mixture, 2 tablespoons cocoa powder, and honey. Blend on high until smooth.

Add the ice cubes and blend on high until thick and smooth.

To serve, pour into 2 glasses and sprinkle with 1/2 teaspoon cocoa powder.

Makes 2 servings.

Berry Good Smoothie

Antioxidant-rich berries are key to a healthful diet. Unfortunately, they have a pretty short growing season. Luckily, this recipe actually works best with frozen berries, so you can enjoy those superfruits even when they're out of season. Kids love this one—maybe because it's bright purple!

- 1/2 cup frozen organic blueberries
- 1/2 cup frozen organic blackberries
- 1/2 cup frozen organic raspberries
- 1/2 cup unsweetened coconut milk
- 2 teaspoons raw honey
- 1/2 teaspoon pure vanilla extract
- 6 ice cubes

In a blender, combine the blueberries, blackberries, raspberries, coconut milk, honey, and vanilla. Blend on high until fairly smooth and consistent in color.

Add the ice cubes and blend on high until thick and creamy.

To serve, pour into 2 tall glasses.

Makes 2 servings.

Creamy Pumpkin Smoothie

This smoothie offers the flavors of fall and pumpkin pie, along with a healthful serving of beta-carotene and fiber, for a perfectly Paleo treat. If you have only a large can of pumpkin puree on hand, the remainder will freeze very well in an airtight container for up to three months; use it in a soup or cake recipe, or another smoothie.

- 3/4 cup pumpkin puree (not pumpkin pie filling)
- 1/2 teaspoon cinnamon, plus extra for garnish
- 1/2 teaspoon ground nutmeg, plus extra for garnish
- 1/4 teaspoon ground cloves
- 1 cup plain, unsweetened almond or coconut milk
- 2 tablespoons pure maple syrup
- 1 teaspoon pure vanilla extract
- 6 ice cubes

In a small bowl, combine the pumpkin puree, cinnamon, nutmeg, and cloves, and stir well with a fork.

In a blender, combine the pumpkin mixture, almond or coconut milk, maple syrup, and vanilla. Blend on high until well mixed.

Add the ice cubes and blend on high until thick and creamy.

To serve, pour into 2 tall glasses and sprinkle with extra cinnamon or nutmeg, if desired.

Makes 2 servings.

PALEO SWEET SNACKS

Chunky Trail Mix

Trail mix becomes a chewy, chunky snack when mixed with honey and baked. It's ready to eat out of hand and much better for you than a candy bar from the office vending machine. It also makes a nutritious topping for your Paleo-style hot cereal.

- 1 teaspoon walnut or coconut oil
- 1 cup raw pecan halves
- 1 cup raw walnut halves
- 1 cup raw pumpkin seeds
- 1 cup unsweetened dried cranberries
- 1 cup unsweetened dried apricots, roughly chopped
- 1/2 cup raw honey
- 1/2 teaspoon sea salt

Preheat oven to 300 degrees F.

Line a 9 x 13–inch glass baking dish with aluminum foil. Grease the foil with the walnut or coconut oil.

In a large mixing bowl, combine the pecans, walnuts, pumpkin seeds, cranberries, and apricots, and stir well.

Microwave the honey for about 45 seconds or until quite thin.

Pour the honey over the nut mixture and quickly stir until evenly incorporated.

Immediately spread the mixture into the baking dish in an even layer, patting down with a spoon. Sprinkle with salt.

Bake for 30 minutes. Let it cool until the trail mix is just warm and is comfortable to handle.

Using your hands or a firm spatula, remove the mixture in large pieces and break into bite-sized chunks. Let it cool completely before storing (it will harden as it cools).

Store in an airtight container for up to 2 weeks.

Makes 5 cups.

Frozen Pineapple Granita

Granita is a fast and easy sorbet that doesn't require an ice-cream maker, and it's the ideal way to use up ripe fruit when it's at peak flavor. It's a refreshing sweet snack or dessert for the whole family on a hot day—and you don't have to turn on your oven!

- 2 cups ripe pineapple, cut in chunks
- 2 tablespoons fresh lemon juice
- 1 cup raw honey

Mint leaves for garnish, if desired

In a blender or food processor, combine the pineapple, lemon juice, and honey. Blend just until smooth.

Pour into a 9 x 13–inch baking dish, cover with plastic wrap, and place on a flat surface in the freezer.

After 30 minutes, stir the mixture thoroughly with a fork and put it back in the freezer.

After another 30 minutes, stir again, then freeze for 1 more hour.

To serve, scoop the granita into ice-cream dishes, and garnish with a fresh mint leaf, if desired.

Makes 4 servings.

Chewy Almond Cookies

Everyone enjoys a chewy cookie, warm and fresh from the oven. This Paleo-friendly recipe allows you to indulge guilt-free. Pour a cold glass of almond or coconut milk and enjoy!

- 1 1/2 cups almond butter
- 2/3 cup raw honey
- 1/2 cup unsweetened applesauce
- 2 large eggs, beaten
- 1/4 cup chopped raw almonds
- 1/2 cup almond flour
- 1/2 teaspoon baking soda
- 1/2 teaspoon cream of tartar
- 1 teaspoon coconut oil

In a large mixing bowl, combine the almond butter, honey, applesauce, eggs, and almonds, and mix well with a spoon.

In a small bowl, combine almond flour, baking soda, and cream of tartar, and mix well with a whisk or fork.

Slowly add the dry ingredients to the wet ingredients, stirring well after each addition.

Cut a 14-inch-long piece of plastic wrap and lay it lengthwise in front of you. Spoon the dough onto the plastic wrap and form a log lengthwise, leaving 1 inch of plastic wrap on either side.

Roll the dough up tightly in the plastic wrap, twist the ends shut, and refrigerate for at least 1 hour.

Preheat oven to 375 degrees F.

Line a baking sheet with aluminum foil and grease the foil with the coconut oil.

Unwrap the dough and cut it into 1/2-inch slices. Place the slices on the baking sheet. (Use additional baking sheets or bake in batches if the cookies don't all fit.)

Bake for 10–11 minutes or until just golden brown. Remove the cookies to a rack to cool.

Store in an airtight container for up to 1 week. These will freeze very well for up to 3 months, either baked or as rolled dough.

Makes about 2 dozen cookies.

Creamy Strawberry Ice Cream

Sometimes, when it's ice cream you want, ice cream you must have—and you can with this Paleo-friendly coconut-based recipe. Organic strawberries are at their best (and least expensive) in summer and fall. Seize that moment to use them fresh in this recipe, and slice and freeze them to enjoy when the season ends.

- 2 (8-ounce) cans unsweetened cream of coconut
- 2 cups unsweetened coconut milk
- Yolks of 6 large eggs, beaten
- Whites of 2 large eggs, beaten
- 1/4 cup raw honey
- 2 tablespoons pure vanilla extract
- 2 cups fresh sliced strawberries, divided

In a blender, combine cream of coconut, coconut milk, egg yolks, egg whites, honey, and vanilla. Blend on low speed until the honey and eggs are fully incorporated.

Add one cup of fresh strawberries to the blender and blend until fairly, but not perfectly, smooth.

Pour into a large bowl and gently stir in the remaining strawberries.

Pour all contents into the bowl of an ice-cream machine, and follow the manufacturer's directions.

Makes 8 servings.

Flourless Cocoa-Mint Cookies

These crispy cookies are light and not overly sweet, so they make an ideal after-dinner treat. They freeze beautifully once baked, so make a double batch to keep on hand for company. They will definitely be impressed.

- 6 large eggs, beaten
- 1/3 cup raw honey
- 1/4 cup plus 1 teaspoon coconut oil, melted
- 1/2 cup cocoa powder
- 1/2 cup unsweetened applesauce
- 1 teaspoon mint extract

Preheat oven to 350 degrees F.

In a large mixing bowl, combine the eggs, honey, and 1/4 cup coconut oil, and stir until well blended.

Whisk in the cocoa powder until there are no dry spots.

Stir in the applesauce and mint extract until just blended.

Line a baking sheet with parchment paper. Grease the parchment with 1 teaspoon coconut oil. Drop the dough by the teaspoon onto the baking sheet.

Bake for 10–12 minutes. They should still be slightly moist at the center.

Slide the parchment paper and cookies off the baking sheet and allow to cool before removing the cookies from the parchment.

Store in an airtight container for up to 1 week, or freeze in a Ziploc-type plastic bag for up to 3 months.

Makes 1 dozen cookies.

Spiced Apple Dip

This dip is perfect alongside crisp, fresh slices of pears, apples, and other firm fruits. Kids love it as a lunch box snack, and everyone will eat it up when served at a buffet or summer party. It's light, fragrant, and just sweet enough. It keeps well, so make it ahead of time and be party-ready!

- 4 sweet apples, such as Jonagold or Golden Delicious
- 1/2 cup almond butter
- 1 teaspoon raw honey
- 1/4 teaspoon ground nutmeg
- 1/2 teaspoon ground cardamom
- 1/4 teaspoon sea salt
- Fresh sliced fruit

Peel, core, and chop the apples, then place them in a food processor or blender. Blend on high until quite smooth.

Add the almond butter, honey, nutmeg, cardamom, and salt, and blend on low until smooth.

Pour the mixture into a small soufflé dish or shallow dip bowl, cover, and refrigerate for at least 2 hours before serving.

To serve, place the dish of dip in the center of a platter and arrange fresh slices of apples, pears, peaches, nectarines, or other seasonal fruit around it.

Store in a tightly covered jar in the refrigerator for up to 1 week.

Makes 2 cups.

Zucchini Bread

This may sound like a savory snack, but it's actually a moist, sweet, quick bread similar to a dense spice cake. Eat it warm on a cool morning or wrap it up for an afternoon pick-me-up. Kids will love it even if they hate zucchini—just don't tell them it's in there! The recipe is for two loaves, because it freezes so well.

- 3 cups coconut flour
- 3 teaspoons baking soda
- 1 teaspoon cinnamon
- 1 teaspoon ground ginger
- 1/2 teaspoon ground cloves
- 1/2 teaspoon cream of tartar
- 1/2 teaspoon sea salt
- 2 cups peeled and grated zucchini, well drained
- 5 large eggs, beaten
- 1 cup unsweetened applesauce
- 1/4 cup raw honey
- 2 tablespoons plus
- 1 teaspoon coconut oil, melted

Preheat oven to 375 degrees F.

In a large mixing bowl, combine the coconut flour, baking soda, cinnamon, ginger, cloves, cream of tartar, and salt, and mix until well blended.

In another large bowl, combine the grated zucchini, eggs, applesauce, honey, and 2 tablespoons coconut oil, and stir with a fork or whisk until well combined.

Add the dry ingredients to the wet mixture 1/2 cup at a time, stirring gently just until there are no dry patches.

Grease two 5 x 9–inch loaf pans with 1 teaspoon coconut oil. Divide the batter between the two pans.

Bake for 45–50 minutes or just until a toothpick inserted in the center comes out clean. Allow to cool in the pans before removing.

Store wrapped in plastic wrap and aluminum foil in the refrigerator for up to 1 week, or in the freezer for up to 3 months.

Makes 2 loaves (about 20 servings).

(6)

LOW-CALORIE PALEO SNACKS

Spiced Kale Chips

Kale chips have become a very popular snack, and not just among Paleo folk. They're a cinch to make and are even more addictive than potato chips (and much lower in calories). They don't keep very well, but it doesn't matter— they'll be long gone before they go stale.

- 2 bunches fresh kale, trimmed and rinsed
- 2 teaspoons light olive oil
- 1/2 teaspoon sea salt
- 1/2 teaspoon freshly ground black pepper
- 1/2 teaspoon paprika
- 1/4 teaspoon ground cumin

Position oven racks at the center and bottom. Preheat oven to 275 degrees F.

Pat the kale thoroughly dry with paper towels or dish towels, then tear the leaves into large pieces. Place in a large bowl.

Pour the olive oil over the kale and toss well to coat (clean hands work best).

Combine the salt, pepper, paprika, and cumin in a small dish, then sprinkle over the kale. Toss again.

Lay the kale out onto two baking sheets, trying not to let the leaves overlap too much.

Bake for 10 minutes, one sheet on the lower rack and one on the center rack.

Flip the leaves carefully with tongs, then switch the positions of the baking sheets. Bake for 10 more minutes or until the leaves are dry and crisp.

Store the chips at room temperature in a Ziploc-type plastic bag for up to 3 days.

Makes 2 servings.

Avocado-Mushroom Bites

This light and fresh take on stuffed mushrooms is the perfect appetizer for a casual dinner party or picnic. If you increase the serving size, they make a nice light lunch or a fun substitute for the same old side salad. Choose an avocado that is just a bit overripe—it'll have the most flavor.

- 16 whole large button mushrooms, stems removed
- 1/2 teaspoon sea salt
- 1/4 teaspoon freshly ground black pepper
- 1 Hass avocado, peeled and mashed (about 3/4 cup)
- 1/4 cup finely chopped red onion
- 1 tablespoon fresh lemon juice
- 1/2 teaspoon ground cumin
- 1/2 teaspoon chili powder

Sprinkle the mushrooms with salt and pepper, then set aside for 15 minutes.

In a medium-sized bowl, combine the avocado, onion, lemon juice, cumin, and chili powder, and stir well.

Using a melon baller or teaspoon, divide the avocado filling among the mushroom caps. Serve immediately.

Makes about 4 appetizer servings.

Pineapple Salsa

This sweet salsa is bursting with freshness and has just enough kick to keep you reaching for more. It tastes even better when its flavors get to mingle in the refrigerator for a couple of days, so it's ideal to make ahead for a party or barbecue.

- 1 cup diced fresh pineapple
- 1 cup diced almost-ripe mango
- 1/2 cup thinly sliced fresh celery
- 1/2 cup diced red onion
- 1 fresh jalapeño pepper, diced (remove seeds for less heat)
- 2 tablespoons fresh lemon juice
- 1 teaspoon chopped fresh cilantro
- 1 teaspoon chopped fresh parsley

In a medium-sized mixing bowl, combine the pineapple, mango, celery, onion, and jalapeño pepper, and stir well.

Pour the lemon juice over all, and stir well.

Add the cilantro and parsley, and stir to combine.

Cover and refrigerate for at least 2 hours or up to 3 days.

Serve the salsa as a dip for fresh vegetables, Paleo-friendly crackers, or even meat jerky.

Makes 3 cups, or about 6 servings.

Spinach and Strawberry Salad with Lemon Vinaigrette

This salad represents the best of summertime freshness. Serve it alongside a bowl of soup for lunch, or enjoy it on its own for a light snack. It's loaded with iron, fiber, and vitamin C, and is one salad that most kids are happy to eat.

For the vinaigrette:

- 1/2 teaspoon grated lemon zest
- 4 tablespoons fresh lemon juice
- 1 teaspoon raw honey
- 4 tablespoons light olive oil
- 1/4 teaspoon sea salt
- 1/4 teaspoon freshly ground black pepper

For the salad:

- 2 cups fresh baby spinach leaves, washed and dried
- 1 cup sliced strawberries

Make the vinaigrette:

In a blender or food processor, combine the lemon zest, lemon juice, and honey, and blend on low speed. Gradually add the oil, and blend until the mixture becomes pale yellow and opaque. Add salt and pepper, and set aside.

Make the salad:

In a medium bowl, combine the spinach leaves and strawberries and toss well.

Divide the salad among four salad plates. Drizzle each portion with vinaigrette, and serve immediately.

Makes 4 servings.

Stuffed Portobello Mushrooms

Portobello mushrooms are meaty, dense, and subtly flavored—perfectly suited to a savory herbed filling. Even meat lovers will enjoy the rich flavor and substantial texture of this dish, which works equally well as a main dish or hearty appetizer.

- 8 portobello mushrooms, brushed clean
- 3 teaspoons olive oil, divided
- 2 stalks celery, finely chopped
- 1 carrot, peeled and grated (about 1/2 cup)
- 1 small yellow onion, diced
- 1/2 cup chopped raw walnuts
- 2 cloves garlic, crushed
- 1/2 teaspoon sea salt
- 1/4 teaspoon freshly ground black pepper
- 1 teaspoon chopped fresh oregano
- 1 teaspoon chopped fresh parsley

Remove the stems from the mushrooms and roughly chop the stems. Set aside.

Pour 1 teaspoon olive oil into a small dish and use your fingers or a pastry brush to coat the outside of each mushroom cap with oil. Place the caps on a baking sheet.

Preheat oven to 350 degrees F.

In a large, heavy skillet, heat 2 teaspoons olive oil over medium heat.

Add the chopped mushroom stems, celery, carrot, onion, walnuts, and garlic, and sauté for 6–8 minutes or until the celery is just tender.

Add the salt, pepper, oregano, and parsley to the pan, and sauté for 1 more minute.

Divide the filling evenly between the mushroom caps, and bake for 12–15 minutes or until the mushrooms are golden brown. Serve warm.

These can be made up to 1 day in advance and reheated when ready to serve.

Makes 4 servings.

Spicy Grilled Summer Fruit

This deceptively simple dish delivers complex flavors with minimum fuss. The recipe calls for a stovetop grill, but you can just as easily use an outdoor grill. Put the fruit in a mesh fish turner if you do use your backyard grill.

- 1 tablespoon light olive oil
- 1/2 teaspoon sea salt
- 1/2 teaspoon freshly ground black pepper
- 1/2 teaspoon mild curry powder

- 8 fresh pineapple rings, about 3/4-inch thick
- 8 wedges fresh cantaloupe, about 1-inch thick (remove the peel)
- 4 fresh nectarines, quartered (unpeeled)

Preheat the stovetop grill over high heat and brush with olive oil.

Combine the salt, pepper, and curry powder, and sprinkle over one side of each piece of fruit.

Arrange the fruit, seasoned side up, on the grill, and cook for 3 minutes.

Use tongs to turn the fruit, and grill for 2 minutes longer.

To serve, arrange a combination of 2 pineapple rings, 2 cantaloupe wedges, and 4 pieces of nectarine onto 4 small plates. Serve warm.

Makes 4 servings.

SECTION TWO
The Basics of the Paleo Diet

7

WHAT IS THE PALEO DIET?

Whether modern health-care professionals want to admit it or not, the Paleo diet closely mirrors what most of them tell their patients: eat more fruits, vegetables, and lean meats, and stay away from processed garbage. The diet, also known as the Stone Age diet, the caveman diet, and the hunter-gatherer diet, has gained a significant following in recent years, and there's some pretty good research to support the switch.

How Did the Paleo Diet Start?

Back in the 1970s a gastroenterologist by the name of Walter L. Voegtlin observed that digestive diseases such as colitis, Crohn's disease, and irritable bowel syndrome were much more prevalent in people who followed a modern Western diet than they were in people's ancestors, whose diet consisted largely of vegetables, fruits, nuts, and lean meats. He began treating patients with these disorders by recommending diets low in carbohydrates and high in animal fats.

Unfortunately, the medical world simply wasn't ready to give up the idea that a low-fat, low-calorie diet was the healthiest way to eat, so

Dr. Voegtlin's observations and research went largely unnoticed, and the Paleo diet was shoved to the back of the drawer.

Finally—The Stone Age Is Cool Again!

Fast-forward a decade to a point when medical researchers had gained considerably more insight into how the human body actually works. Melvin Konner, S. Boyd Eaton, and Marjorie Shostak of Emory University published a book called *The Paleolithic Prescription: A Program of Diet and Exercise and a Design for Living*, then followed it up with a second book, *The Stone-Age Health Programme: Diet and Exercise as Nature Intended*. The first book became the foundation for most of the modern versions of the Paleo diet, and the second backed it up with more research.

The main difference was that instead of eliminating any foods that people's ancestors wouldn't have had access to as Dr. Voegtlin did originally, Konner, Eaton, and Shostak encouraged eating foods that were nutritionally and proportionally similar to a traditional caveman diet. Because it was more realistic, the diet caught on like wildfire, and the research in favor of it continues to grow.

What Are the Rules?

Paleo is one of the easiest diets on the planet to follow: just remember to keep it real. If it's processed, artificial, or otherwise not directly from the earth, don't eat it. It's that simple. Here's a list of the delicious, healthful foods that the Paleo diet encourages:

- Eggs
- Healthful oils—olive and coconut are best; canola oil is under debate right now, too
- Lean animal proteins
- Nuts and seeds (note, however, that peanuts are NOT nuts)

- Organic fruits
- Organic vegetables
- Seafood, especially cold-water fish such as salmon and tuna in order to get the most omega-3 fatty acids

Sounds kind of familiar, doesn't it? That's because it's probably what your doctor encouraged you to eat more of the last time that you went to see him or her! Now let's take a look at some foods that are off the table if you're going to eat Stone Age style:

- Alcohol
- Artificial foods, such as preservatives and zero-calorie sweeteners
- Cereal grains, such as wheat, barley, hops, corn, oats, rye, and rice
- Dairy (though some followers allow dairy for the health benefits)
- Legumes (including peanuts)
- Processed foods, such as wheat flour and sugar
- Processed meats, such as bacon, deli meats, sausage, and canned meats
- Starchy vegetables (though these are currently under debate)

Frequently Asked Questions

Now that you have a general idea of what you can and can't eat, you may still have a few questions, so here's a list of those most frequently asked.

Q. Why do I have to quit drinking?

A. Beer is basically liquid grain, and it's packed with empty calories. Many types of alcoholic products contain gluten, which is discussed in detail in Chapter 9. Mixed drinks and wine are often loaded with sugar. If you absolutely can't go without that Friday-night cocktail, shoot for red wine, tequila, potato vodka, or white rum—and be careful what you mix it with.

Q. Why are legumes forbidden? They're natural foods and great sources of protein.

A. Most legumes, in their raw state, are toxic. They contain lectins—proteins that bind carbohydrates and have been shown to cause such autoimmune diseases as lupus and rheumatoid arthritis. The phytates in many legumes inhibit your absorption of critical minerals, and the protease inhibitors interfere with how your body breaks down protein.

Q. Why no dairy?

A. This one's under debate and there are many Paleo followers who still incorporate dairy regularly into their diets. The main reason that dairy is generally forbidden is that humans are the only animals who drink milk as adults, and many food allergies and digestive disorders are lactose related. There's a much more scientific answer for this question, but it boils down to believing or not believing that milk is bad for you.

Q. How will I lose weight eating fat?

A. This is a question that most people have initially because you're programmed to believe that red meat is bad for your heart. The fact is lean, organic, free-range meat is an excellent source of protein and many other vitamins and minerals. You're not going to be living on it alone; you're going to be incorporating it into a healthful diet.

Q. Peanuts are nuts and corn is a vegetable, so why are they off-limits?

A. *Au contraire.* Peanuts are legumes and corn is a grain. Be careful that you know what food groups everything you eat falls into or you may sabotage your efforts to be healthier.

(8)

THE BENEFITS OF PALEO

Many people turn to the Paleo diet because of the weight-loss benefits, but that's not where the idea originated. If you remember, the diet was created by a gastroenterologist to help his patients with various gastric disorders. Of course, weight loss is a wonderful side effect that has its own set of healthful benefits.

When you add in the myriad other perks, going caveman is almost a no-brainer. Let's take a quick peek at some of the biggest health benefits of following a Paleo diet.

Weight Loss

Since this is one of the primary reasons that many people decide to switch to a Paleo diet, this is a good place to start. Because you're eliminating empty carbs and adding in lots of healthful plant fiber and lean protein, losing weight will be much easier. A few other factors that contribute to healthful weight loss include:

- Plant fiber takes longer to digest, so you feel full longer.
- Lean proteins help keep your energy levels steady while you build muscle.

- Omega-3s help boost your metabolism and reduce body fat.
- You'll be eating a greater volume of food but taking in fewer calories.

The bottom line is that you'll be consuming foods that help your body function the way that it's supposed to, and one of the natural side effects of that is weight loss.

Healthy Digestive System

Remember that this was the original reason for the diet to be utilized. The theory is that people's bodies aren't adapted to eating grains, dairy, and other foods that are forbidden by the Paleo diet, and so they cause digestive upset, inflammation, and discomfort. Also, your digestive tract needs fiber to help it sweep food through your system or else it builds up and causes problems. Just some of the conditions that may be improved by going caveman include:

- Colitis
- Constipation
- Gas
- Heartburn
- Irritable bowel syndrome

Many people who begin the Paleo diet for other reasons, such as weight loss or heart health, report improved digestive health. Yet another reason that this incredible diet is worth your time!

Type 2 Diabetes Prevention

In the United States and other cultures that have adopted a Western diet, type 2 diabetes has reached disastrous proportions. Historically an adult disease, children are developing this debilitating illness at an alarming rate, and there's no sign of this trend changing. One of the main culprits is excess consumption of processed sugars and flours.

By simply eliminating these calorie-laden, nutritionless foods from your diet, you can literally save your own life. The Paleo diet helps you avoid type 2 diabetes as well as metabolic syndrome, a precursor to many different diseases, for the following reasons:

- Omega-3s help reduce belly fat, an indicator of diabetes and metabolic syndrome.
- Lean proteins and plant fiber help increase insulin resistance so that your sugar levels don't spike.
- The vitamin C that's so readily available in citrus fruits and colorful veggies helps reduce belly fat.
- Lean protein takes longer to metabolize so you avoid energy highs and lows.

Immune Health

When you eat foods that your body isn't adapted to, such as processed grains, legumes, and dairy products, your body produces an allergic response in the form of inflammation, even if you don't experience any obvious outward symptoms. You may notice dark circles under your eyes as well as a feeling of general lethargy. You may attribute these symptoms to stress or exhaustion, but they're actually signs of a chronic allergy.

Inflammation in your body is a bad thing if it's occurring chronically, and it has been causally linked to such autoimmune disorders as:

- Fibromyalgia
- Lupus
- Multiple sclerosis
- Rheumatoid arthritis
- Several different types of cancer

The sad part here is that you don't even realize what you're doing to your body because there are often no symptoms until you have developed the disease. Switching to the Paleo diet may help reduce or eliminate your risk of many debilitating illnesses.

Cardiovascular Health

For most of your life, you've probably been told how horrible red meat and other animal proteins are for your heart, but recent research indicates that this is simply not true. Remember that there's a huge difference in scarfing down a fatty hamburger or sausage and enjoying a lean, organic, grass-fed steak. The burger and sausage are full of saturated fats and, most likely, hormones and additives.

On the other hand, steak is a lean, nutritious protein that delivers essential vitamins and minerals with very little bad fat and no empty calories, preservatives, or hormones. When you throw omega-3s and LDL-lowering healthful fats into the mix, you've got a heart-healthful meal that's good for anybody.

A Few Final Words on Health

The health benefits of giving up processed flour, refined sugar, and foods that cause inflammatory responses could fill an entire doctoral thesis, and the advantages to eliminating hormones and artificial additives from foods could fill another one. This chapter didn't even touch on how a Paleo diet can help with allergies, cancer, brain health, joint health, or celiac disease, but some of these will be covered in the discussion of the health risks of gluten in the next chapter. Suffice to say, the benefits of going Paleo far outweigh the relatively minor inconvenience of giving up a few foods.

9

THE TROUBLE WITH GLUTEN

Of the many health benefits of switching to a Paleo diet, one of the main benefits is that foods allowed on the diet don't have gluten in them. For millions of people worldwide, eating caveman-style is a relatively simple way to avoid digestive upset and even cancers that are caused by an allergy to gluten.

What Is Gluten?

Latin for "glue," gluten is a protein found in wheat and grains that gives the ground flours elasticity and helps them to rise. It's also the binding component that gives bread its chewy texture and keeps it from crumbling apart after baking. Because gluten is insoluble in water, it can be removed from flour, but typically when you do that, you lose all of the good properties that make breads and cakes what they are.

Without gluten, your baked goods won't rise and they'll have a grainy, crumbly texture. They won't taste anything like their gluten-laden cousins, and you probably won't want to eat more after the first bite. Because of an increasing demand for gluten-free products, food corporations have dedicated a tremendous amount of time and money into creating tasty, effective gluten-free products. Unfortunately, most commercially prepared gluten-free recipe mixes still fall short.

Is the Paleo Diet Gluten-Free?

Because gluten naturally occurs in wheat and grains, the Paleo diet is completely gluten-free. All grain products are strictly forbidden. Remember, the original creator of the diet was a gastroenterologist developing a plan that would help his patients with gastric disorders. Gluten intolerance is one of the most prevalent causes of gastrointestinal distress in Western civilization.

What Is Gluten Intolerance?

Gluten intolerance, or celiac disease in its advanced stage, is a condition that damages the small intestine, and it's triggered by eating foods that have gluten in them. Some of these foods include:

- Bread
- Cookies
- Just about any baked goods
- Most flours, including white and wheat flours
- Pasta
- Pizza dough

Gluten triggers an immune response in the small intestine that causes damage to its inside. This can lead to an inability to absorb vital nutrients. Other illnesses associated with this disease include lactose intolerance, bone loss, several types of cancer, neurological complications, and malnutrition. Diseases notwithstanding, just the symptoms of gluten intolerance can disrupt daily life. They include:

- Depression
- Fatigue
- Joint pain
- Neuropathy
- Osteoporosis
- Rashes
- Severe diarrhea
- Stomach cramps

These are only a few of the symptoms that a person with gluten intolerance can suffer from, and since all foods that contain gluten are forbidden on the Paleo diet, you can see what the appeal is.

The Harmful Effects of Gluten

Gluten doesn't just harm people with fully developed celiac disease. It's actually harmful to everyone. Long-term studies indicate that people who have even a mild sensitivity to gluten exhibit a significantly higher risk of death than people who do not. The worst part is that 99 percent of people with gluten sensitivity don't even know they have it. They attribute their symptoms to other conditions, such as stress or fatigue.

Absorption Malfunction

One of the attributes that many obese or overweight people share is the fact that they can still feel hungry after eating a full meal. This feeling of hunger is because gluten sensitivity is preventing your body from absorbing vital nutrients.

Food Addiction

There are chemicals called exorphins in some foods that cause you to crave food even when you're not hungry. Food addiction is a serious issue and doesn't necessarily denote a lack of willpower; these exorphins are actually a drug-like chemical released in your brain that creates an irresistible desire for more food. Gluten contains as many as fifteen different exorphins.

Though food companies have created gluten-free foods, they often replace the gluten with flavor-enhancers, such as sodium and sugar, which can still seriously sabotage your dieting and fitness efforts. Another advantage to the Paleo diet is that by following it, you're not only eliminating gluten, you're also avoiding the pitfalls of commercially prepared foods that continue to make you sick.

Other Conditions Related to Gluten

There are numerous other conditions related to gluten sensitivity, and many professionals postulate that this is simply because people's bodies aren't adapted to eating grains so they are treated as allergens. Other symptoms or disorders linked to eating gluten include:

- Anxiety
- Autism
- Dementia
- Migraines
- Mouth sores
- Schizophrenia
- Seizures

These aren't just minor aches and pains, though gluten sensitivity can cause those, too. These are major diseases and conditions that can ruin your life. It's no wonder that people who know that they suffer from gluten intolerance consider the Paleo diet.

Health Benefits of Going Gluten-Free

Obviously, there are countless benefits of giving up gluten, but here are a few that may be of particular interest to you:

- Decreased chance of several types of cancer
- Healthy, painless digestion
- Healthy skin
- Improved brain function
- Improved mood
- Reduced appetite
- Weight loss (or gain, if you're underweight because of malnutrition)

With the obvious advantages of giving up grains, it's difficult to understand exactly why people would hesitate. It's just a matter of making some adjustments to your diet, and now that understanding about both food and health is increasing, there are some great alternatives out there that will help you get rid of your addiction to grains!

⑩

PALEO FOOD GUIDE

Shopping for foods that are Paleo friendly can be a daunting task when you're first starting out. What's allowed and what's not? What are all of those mystery ingredients that are listed in foods? For the most part, stocking your fridge and pantry is fairly simple, but there are going to be times when you don't want to eat just steak and broccoli, and there will be other times when you need something fast and simple. Don't worry: you'll get the hang of it.

There are a few different versions of the Paleo diet, but this discussion will focus on the modern middle road so that it's easier for you to make the transition to your new, healthier lifestyle. Throughout the following paragraphs, you'll learn what foods are OK and where you can find them. You'll also learn some alternate ingredients for baking muffins and other goodies that won't get you kicked out of the cave!

Paleo Pantry and Kitchen Tips

The first bit of good news is that you're not going to be counting calories. Instead, you're going to try to keep your portions in line with what your ancestors most likely ate. A diet that consists of 50 to 60 percent protein, 30 to 45 percent healthful carbs, and 5 to 10 percent healthful vegetable fats, such as olive oil, avocados, nuts, and seeds, is the general goal.

Basically, when you're stacking your plate, put your protein on one side and your fruits and veggies on the other. Snacks can be whatever you want, but veggies and nuts are great choices. Be careful with nuts and fruits; though they're good for you, they're high in calories and can sabotage your weight-loss efforts if you're not careful.

If Possible, Go Raw

Many fruits and vegetables lose nutritional value when you cook them, so when possible, eat them raw. You'll also eat less because you'll be chewing more. If you opt to cook your veggies, steam them lightly so they maintain their bright colors. A key clue that you've cooked your greens to death is that they've lost that pretty vibrant green hue and turned an olive color. Try to avoid that.

Steaming, baking, grilling, and broiling are all great methods of cooking and require little added fat to prevent sticking. It should go without saying that the fryer can be retired to the garage to be sold at your next rummage sale.

Cooking on the Fly

Meals away from home can be a real challenge when you're first starting out. Restaurants are filled with tempting burgers and fries, and you have no idea what's in the salad dressings. If you must eat out, order a plain garden salad with oil and vinegar. You could also request a steak or chicken breast to go on top, but make sure that they either grill it dry or use olive oil.

Opt not to eat out in the beginning. Instead, make an amazing soup at home for dinner with enough leftover that you aren't tempted to go out for a quick fix. That way, you know what's in your food and you know that it's going to be delicious!

Plan Ahead

If you know in advance what you're going to eat for lunch or for dinner, you're not going to be as likely to cheat with something quick from the vending machine. Take snacks to work with you so that the box of doughnuts isn't so tempting.

Meats and Proteins

Your meats need to come from grass-fed, organic livestock, free-range poultry, or wild-caught fish and seafood. Wild game is great, too, if you're so inclined. Actually, meats such as venison are extremely low in bad fats and high in good fats and lean protein, so feel free to partake!

Fruits and Vegetables

If at all possible, shop at your local farmers' market for fresh organic fruits and veggies. Since the Paleo diet is dependent upon your creativity to complete a hot, fresh, delicious meal without the aid of flours, fats, and no-no's, you're going to have to learn a number of ways to prepare dishes. Plus, if you're offering a wide variety of foods that your family knows and loves, you won't be under so much pressure to create a single main dish that everybody will eat and enjoy.

Tomatoes are a great addition to any salad and make a flavorful base for soups and sauces. They're packed with nutrients and have so many uses that you should always have some on hand. Other staples should include carrots, peppers, cauliflower, and celery.

For fruits, opt for ones that are high in nutrients and relatively low in sugar, such as stone fruits and berries. Berries are also fabulous sources of antioxidants, phytonutrients, and vitamins. Apples are an easy grab-and-go food, as are peaches, oranges, and bananas. The dark tip of the banana that you usually pick off is rich in vitamin K, so eat it!

Oils and Fats

Oils high in saturated fats, such as corn oil and vegetable oil, are out. Opt instead for oils that are high in omega-3s, such as olive oil, avocado oil, coconut oil, and possibly canola oil. The latter is currently a point of contention among long-term Paleo followers, but there's a compelling argument to include it.

Seasonings

Your success with making the transition to the caveman way of eating is largely dependent on how flavorful your food is. As a result, you're going to need to incorporate various herbs and spices to make your dishes delicious. Here are a few that you should always have on hand:

- Allspice
- Black pepper
- Basil
- Cayenne pepper
- Cinnamon
- Cloves
- Crushed red pepper
- Curry powder
- Dry mustard
- Garlic—fresh and powdered
- Mustard seed
- Oregano
- Paprika
- Parsley
- Rosemary
- Thyme

Snacks

Finally, you'll probably want to keep some snacks on hand. Now, that does NOT mean cupcakes, potato chips, or crackers. However, there are still many options, such as certain beef jerky (or even better, make your own!), dried fruits, nuts, and seeds. They're satisfying and add nutrients to your diet instead of unhealthful fats.

Paleo Shopping Tips

Going to the grocery store is going to be a bit of a challenge at first, just as it is anytime that you make changes to your diet. Especially if you're accustomed to eating a large amount of refined flour and sugar and aren't yet over your sugar addiction, it's not going to be easy. Here are a few tips to help you along your way.

- Shop for your produce at the local farmers' market if possible.
- When at the grocery store, shop around the perimeter of the store. That's where most stores keep all of their meats and produce, and 99 percent of your food is going to come from those departments. If you need to get something from an aisle, go straight in, get it, and get back to the perimeter before those cookies catch your eye!
- Make a list and stick to it.
- If you do choose to eat canned fruits and veggies, make sure that you read the label so that you're not getting hidden sodium and preservatives.
- Buy meat in bulk when you catch a sale.
- Don't shop hungry! Have a low-fat, high-protein snack before you go so that you aren't tempted while you're there.

CONCLUSION

M any people, especially those new to the Paleo diet, tend to become so focused on what they *can't eat* that they lose sight of all the wonderful fresh foods that are encouraged in the Paleo lifestyle.

There is a huge variety of delicious ingredients just waiting to be made into exciting and tempting snacks and treats. Experiment with at least one new ingredient and one new recipe per week, and you'll soon have an arsenal of tried-and-true favorites.

With all of the sweet and savory possibilities available to you, you can have enough snacks, desserts, and treats to feed a small army of children, a hungry bunch of football fans, or a grazing teenager without ever having to fall into a rut.

Kids are easy to win over to Paleo eating when you fill their lunch boxes and snack plates with colorful, varied ingredients and healthful, Paleo-friendly versions of junk food favorites. There is a huge array of recipes out there for baked goods, such as cookies, snack bars, and muffins, that will satisfy a kid's sweet tooth and make parents happy, too. For more fun, delicious recipes, try *Paleo Cookies: Gluten-Free Paleo Cookie Recipes for a Paleo Diet* and *Paleo Muffins: Gluten-Free Paleo Muffin Recipes for a Paleo Diet.*

Eating Paleo is all about learning to love whole, nutritious foods and then enjoying the way eating them makes you feel. Food should be savored and shared, and Paleo foods are no exception.

Try out these Paleo-friendly snack recipes, discover and create your own, and make the most of your healthful Paleo diet!